FREEDOM FROM SICKLE CELL DISEASE

DIVINE MEDICINE THAT IS EFFECTIVE

BY
IHEKE WILLIAMS

Unless otherwise indicated, all scripture quotations are taken from the King James Version of the Bible A key for other Bible versions used;

NKJV	New King James Version
AMP	The Amplified Bible
TANT	The New Amplified Bible
TLB -	The Living Bible
CEV -	Contemporary English Version
NASB	New American Standard Version
GW -	God's Word version
ESV -	English Standard Version
NET -	New English Translation
ISV -	International Standard Version
NIV -	New International Version
MSG -	The Message Translation

DEDICATION

This Book is dedicated to Almighty God and to everyone in the world.

TABLE OF CONTENT

WHAT IS SICKLE CELL DISEASE?

Sickle Cell disease is a group of blood disorders typically inherited from a person's parents. The most common type is known as sickle cell anaemia (SCA).

Sickle cell disease occurs when a person inherits two abnormal copies of the haemoglobin gene, one from each parent.

Source: Wikipedia

WHAT IS GOD'S SOLUTION

But He was wounded for our transgressions, he was bruised for our iniquities: the chastisement of our peace was upon Him; and with His stripes we are healed – Isaiah 53:5 (KJV)

"...By His wounds ye have been healed" - 1 Peter 2:24 (KJV)

The phrase "...ye HAVE BEEN HEALED" is in the past tense, it means JESUS has ALREADY HEALED you from Sickle cell disease, years ago.

You have NO business with sickle cell disease anymore. YOU ARE FREE!!

You are Healed already: FREE and ACTIVE Forever because of the sufferings of Christ on the cross for your sake.

For the next 31 days and forever, you will affirm this blessing that Our Lord Jesus Christ has given to you and you will you live in perfect health FOREVER!.

INSTRUCTION 1

That if thou shalt <u>confess with thy mouth</u> the Lord Jesus, and shalt <u>believe in thine heart</u> that God hath raised him from the dead, thou shalt be saved. – Romans 10:9

We having the same <u>spirit of faith</u>, according as it is written, I believed, and therefore have I spoken; <u>we also believe, and therefore speak</u>; - 2 Corinthians 4:13

There has to be a connection with what you say/affirm with your mouth and what you have in your heart or what you believe in your heart.

Consequently, for the affirmations to be effective, you will have to meditate on the scripture (1 Peter 2:24) for 5 minutes, in your heart, before you affirm it with your mouth.

Don't say anything to the contrary during the period of affirmations.

INSTRUCTION 2

"For our light affliction, which is but for a moment, worketh for us a far more exceeding and eternal weight of glory;

While we look not at the things which are seen, but at the things which are not seen: for the things which are seen are temporal; but the things which are not seen are eternal. – 2 Corinthians 4:17-18 (KJV)

For the duration of the affirmations, do not touch any part of your body that might have been affected by this sickness. If it is possible, don't look at it.

The word of God (1 Peter 2:24) in your heart will not be effective when you keep recognizing the presence of a sickness because doubt will begin to develop in your heart and the word doesn't work in the presence of doubts/unbelief.

Follow these instructions, **BE CONSISTENT** and your affirmations will be very effective.

DAY 1
AFFIRMATION

Meditate on 1 Peter 2:24B in your heart for 5 minutes

"..By His stripes ye have been healed"

Now affirm this BLESSING

"I HAVE BEEN HEALED THEREFORE, I AFFIRM THAT THERE IS NO SICKLE CELL DISEASE INSIDE ME!"

DAY 2
AFFIRMATION

Meditate on 1 Peter 2:24B in your heart for 5 minutes

"..By His stripes ye have been healed"

Now affirm this BLESSING

"I HAVE BEEN HEALED THEREFORE, I AFFIRM THAT I AM ACTIVE AND STRONG FOREVER!"

DAY 3
AFFIRMATION

Meditate on 1 Peter 2:24B in your heart for 5 minutes

"..By His stripes ye have been healed"

Now affirm this BLESSING

"I HAVE BEEN HEALED THEREFORE, I AFFIRM THAT MY IMMUNE SYSTEM IS ACTIVE AND STRONG FOREVER!"

DAY 4
AFFIRMATION

Meditate on 1 Peter 2:24B in your heart for 5 minutes

"..By His stripes ye have been healed"

Now affirm this BLESSING

"I HAVE BEEN HEALED THEREFORE, I AFFIRM THAT I AM ACTIVE AND STRONG FOREVER!"

DAY 5
AFFIRMATION

Meditate on 1 Peter 2:24B in
your heart for 5 minutes

"..By His stripes ye have been
healed"

Now affirm this BLESSING

"I HAVE BEEN HEALED THEREFORE, I AFFIRM THAT THERE IS NO SICKLE CELL DISEASE INSIDE ME!"

DAY 6
AFFIRMATION

Meditate on 1 Peter 2:24B in your heart for 5 minutes

"..By His stripes ye have been healed"

Now affirm this BLESSING

"I HAVE BEEN HEALED THEREFORE, I AFFIRM THAT I AM ACTIVE AND STRONG FOREVER!"

DAY 7
AFFIRMATION

Meditate on 1 Peter 2:24B in your heart for 5 minutes

"..By His stripes ye have been healed"

Now affirm this BLESSING

"I HAVE BEEN HEALED THEREFORE, I AFFIRM THAT THERE IS NO SICKLE CELL DISEASE INSIDE ME!"

DAY 8
AFFIRMATION

Meditate on 1 Peter 2:24B in
your heart for 5 minutes

"..By His stripes ye have been
healed"

Now affirm this BLESSING

"I HAVE BEEN HEALED THEREFORE, I AFFIRM THAT I AM ACTIVE AND STRONG FOREVER!"

DAY 9
AFFIRMATION

Meditate on 1 Peter 2:24B in your heart for 5 minutes

"..By His stripes ye have been healed"

Now affirm this BLESSING

"I HAVE BEEN HEALED THEREFORE, I AFFIRM THAT THERE IS NO SICKLE CELL DISEASE INSIDE ME!"

AFFIRMATION

Meditate on 1 Peter 2:24B in your heart for 5 minutes

"..By His stripes ye have been healed"

Now affirm this BLESSING

"I HAVE BEEN HEALED THEREFORE, I AFFIRM THAT I AM ACTIVE AND STRONG FOREVER!"

Meditate on 1 Peter 2:24B in your heart for 5 minutes

"..By His stripes ye have been healed"

Now affirm this BLESSING

"I HAVE BEEN HEALED THEREFORE, I AFFIRM THAT THERE IS NO SICKLE CELL DISEASE INSIDE ME !"

DAY 12
AFFIRMATION

Meditate on 1 Peter 2:24B in your heart for 5 minutes

"..By His stripes ye have been healed"

Now affirm this BLESSING

"I HAVE BEEN HEALED THEREFORE, I AFFIRM THAT I AM ACTIVE AND STRONG FOREVER!"

DAY 13
AFFIRMATION

Meditate on 1 Peter 2:24B in
your heart for 5 minutes

"..By His stripes ye have been
healed"

Now affirm this BLESSING

"I HAVE BEEN HEALED THEREFORE, I AFFIRM THAT THERE IS NO SICKLE CELL DISEASE INSIDE ME!"

AFFIRMATION

Meditate on 1 Peter 2:24B in your heart for 5 minutes

"..By His stripes ye have been healed"

Now affirm this BLESSING

"I HAVE BEEN HEALED THEREFORE, I AFFIRM THAT I AM ACTIVE AND STRONG FOREVER!"

Meditate on 1 Peter 2:24B in your heart for 5 minutes

"..By His stripes ye have been healed"

Now affirm this BLESSING

"I HAVE BEEN HEALED THEREFORE, I AFFIRM THAT THERE IS NO SICKLE CELL DISEASE INSIDE ME!"

Meditate on 1 Peter 2:24B in your heart for 5 minutes

"..By His stripes ye have been healed"

Now affirm this BLESSING

"I HAVE BEEN HEALED THEREFORE, I AFFIRM THAT I AM ACTIVE AND STRONG FOREVER !"

DAY 17
AFFIRMATION

Meditate on 1 Peter 2:24B in
your heart for 5 minutes

"..By His stripes ye have been
healed"

Now affirm this BLESSING

"I HAVE BEEN HEALED THEREFORE, I AFFIRM THAT THERE IS NO SICKLE CELL DISEASE INSIDE ME !"

DAY 18
AFFIRMATION

Meditate on 1 Peter 2:24B in your heart for 5 minutes

" ..By His stripes ye have been healed"

Now affirm this BLESSING

"I HAVE BEEN HEALED THEREFORE, I AFFIRM THAT I AM ACTIVE AND STRONG FOREVER !"

Meditate on 1 Peter 2:24B in your heart for 5 minutes

"..By His stripes ye have been healed"

Now affirm this BLESSING

"I HAVE BEEN HEALED THEREFORE, I AFFIRM THAT THERE IS NO SICKLE CELL DISEASE INSIDE ME!"

DAY 20
AFFIRMATION

Meditate on 1 Peter 2:24B in your heart for 5 minutes

"..By His stripes ye have been healed"

Now affirm this BLESSING

"I HAVE BEEN HEALED THEREFORE, I AFFIRM THAT I AM ACTIVE AND STRONG FOREVER!"

DAY 21
AFFIRMATION

Meditate on 1 Peter 2:24B in
your heart for 5 minutes

"..By His stripes ye have been
healed"

Now affirm this BLESSING

"I HAVE BEEN HEALED THEREFORE, I AFFIRM THAT THERE IS NO SICKLE CELL DISEASE INSIDE ME!"

<u>AFFIRMATION</u>

Meditate on 1 Peter 2:24B in your heart for 5 minutes

"..By His stripes ye have been healed"

Now affirm this BLESSING

"I HAVE BEEN HEALED THEREFORE, I AFFIRM THAT I AM ACTIVE AND STRONG FOREVER!"

Meditate on 1 Peter 2:24B in
your heart for 5 minutes

" ..By His stripes ye have been
healed"

Now affirm this BLESSING

"I HAVE BEEN HEALED THEREFORE, I AFFIRM THAT THERE IS NO SICKLE CELL DISEASE INSIDE ME !"

DAY 24
AFFIRMATION

Meditate on 1 Peter 2:24B in your heart for 5 minutes

" ..By His stripes ye have been healed"

Now affirm this BLESSING

"I HAVE BEEN HEALED THEREFORE, I AFFIRM THAT I AM ACTIVE AND STRONG FOREVER!"

DAY 25
AFFIRMATION

Meditate on 1 Peter 2:24B in
your heart for 5 minutes

"..By His stripes ye have been
healed"

Now affirm this BLESSING

"I HAVE BEEN HEALED THEREFORE, I AFFIRM THAT THERE IS NO SICKLE CELL DISEASE INSIDE ME!"

DAY 26
AFFIRMATION

Meditate on 1 Peter 2:24B in your heart for 5 minutes

" ..By His stripes ye have been healed"

Now affirm this BLESSING

"I HAVE BEEN HEALED THEREFORE, I AFFIRM THAT I AM ACTIVE AND STRONG FOREVER!"

DAY 27
AFFIRMATION

Meditate on 1 Peter 2:24B in
your heart for 5 minutes

"..By His stripes ye have been
healed"

Now affirm this BLESSING

"I HAVE BEEN HEALED THEREFORE, I AFFIRM THAT THERE IS NO SICKLE CELL DISEASE INSIDE ME!"

DAY 28
AFFIRMATION

Meditate on 1 Peter 2:24B in your heart for 5 minutes

"..By His stripes ye have been healed"

Now affirm this BLESSING

"I HAVE BEEN HEALED THEREFORE, I AFFIRM THAT I AM ACTIVE AND STRONG FOREVER!"

DAY 29
AFFIRMATION

Meditate on 1 Peter 2:24B in your heart for 5 minutes

"..By His stripes ye have been healed"

Now affirm this BLESSING

"I HAVE BEEN HEALED THEREFORE, I AFFIRM THAT THERE IS NO SICKLE CELL DISEASE INSIDE ME!"

DAY 30
AFFIRMATION

Meditate on 1 Peter 2:24B in your heart for 5 minutes

" ..By His stripes ye have been healed"

Now affirm this BLESSING

"I HAVE BEEN HEALED THEREFORE, I AFFIRM THAT I AM ACTIVE AND STRONG FOREVER!"

DAY 31
AFFIRMATION

Meditate on 1 Peter 2:24B in your heart for 5 minutes

"..By His stripes ye have been healed"

Now affirm this BLESSING

"I HAVE BEEN HEALED THEREFORE, I AFFIRM THAT I AM ACTIVE AND STRONG FOREVER!"

"..by His stripes ye
__HAVE BEEN HEALED__"-
1 PETER 2:24

Jesus Christ has paid the price for your peace. Don't let Satan deceive you that you are sick.

Don't let Satan put you in bondage any longer.

Your body has been healed already. You have NO business with sickness.

You are ACTIVE AND STRONG FOREVER!

You are FREE FOREVER!

PRAYER FOR SALVATION

We believe that you have been blessed and that you want to receive eternal life that God has made available to everyone who believes in his love and his grace which He expressed lavishly through His Son Jesus Christ.

"For God so loved the world, that He gave his only begotten Son, that whosoever <u>believeth</u> in him should not perish, but <u>have everlasting life</u>." - John 3:16

Say this prayer to God and believe it with your heart

"Father, I believe that you gave me your only Son to die for my sin. I believe you raised Him from the dead. I declare that your son, Jesus Christ is the Lord of my life. I receive eternal life and I receive the Holy Spirit. I am saved forever.in Jesus name. I am so Happy that today and forever, I am your child. Amen ".

Congratulations, you are now a child of God Halleluyah!! – John 1:12

OTHER INFORMATION

Please share your testimonies via the following handles;

ihekewilliams@gmail.com
+2348061530541

Other Books written by the author includes

Dad, Pray for your Daughter
Mum, Pray for your Daughter
Mum, pray for your Son
Don't stop the flow of the Blessing
Daddy's Prayers
Mummy's Prayers
Divine Health Affirmations Against Infertility
Divine Health Affirmation Against HIV
Divine Health Affirmation Series
FREEDOM SERIES
https://www.amazon.com/Iheke-w.-Okpara/e/B01KFYO1PU/ref=ntt_dp_epwbk_0

ABOUT THE AUTHOR

Iheke Williams is a firm follower and disciple of the Lord Jesus Christ. He is a passionate minister of the grace of our Lord and savior Jesus Christ and has brought the reality of the divine life of Christ into the lives of so many.

Iheke Williams has a calling to communicate the gospel of Christ with simplicity and to show the world how to activate the eternal life of God that is in us already which includes Divine health, Divine righteousness, Divine security and Divine prosperity.

As you read this book and other books written by Iheke Williams you will literally begin to function and manifest the life of God that is already inside you to the glory of God the Father who is the author of all grace and mercy. Amen!

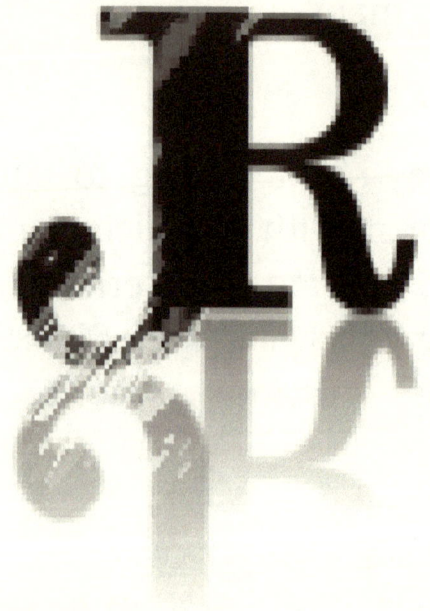

"..by His stripes ye
HAVE BEEN HEALED"-
1 PETER 2:24

You are
FREE
FOREVER!!